I0187834

CONGRATULATIONS ON YOUR DECISION TO GET HEALTHY!

"All Natural Soups & Stews"

COOKBOOK IX

A guide to a *new healthy "comfort food" slow cooker recipe plan* that is not a "DIET", created based on personal experience to help you *finally* keep up with your weight loss management, weight management and overall health goals.

ALSO BY KYLA LATRICE, MBA

"ALL NATURAL SOUPS & STEWS"

A NATURAL SOUPS & STEWS RECIPE GUIDE
for those whom want to maintain good health, lose weight,
maintain weight, fight obesity and/or have a *variety* of healthy
meals to make throughout their lives

KYLA LATRICE, MBA

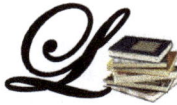

Lady Mirage Publications, Inc.

New York   Memphis   Los Angeles   London   Cape Town   Toronto
Atlanta   Singapore   Japan

Copyright © 2014 by Ms. Kyla Latrice, Inc.
The author is represented by Lady Mirage Literary Agency, Inc.
All rights reserved. In accordance with the U.S. Copyright Act of
1976, the scanning, uploading, and electronic sharing of any part of
this book without the permission of the publisher is unlawful piracy
and theft of the author's intellectual property. If you would like to
use material from the book (other than for review purposes), prior
written permission must be obtained by contacting the publisher at
www.LadyMirageAgency.com
Thank you for your support of the author's rights.

Published by:
Lady Mirage Publications, Inc.
3724 Goodman Rd W, Unit 575
Horn Lake, MS 38637
www.LadyMirageAgency.com

Manufactured in the United States of America
First Edition: November 2014

Lady Mirage Publications, Inc. is an imprint and subsidiary
of Lady Mirage Global. The Lady Mirage Publications, Inc. name
and logo are trademarks of Lady Mirage Global.

Authors within the Lady Mirage Global (under Lady Mirage Agency,
Inc.), Lady Mirage Publications and Lady Mirage Literary Agency
speakers division provides a wide range of authors for speaking
engagements. To find out more information, go to
www.LadyMirageAgency.com
Cover photos provided by www.FreeDigitalPhotos.net
The publisher is not responsible for websites (or their content) that
are not owned by the publisher.

Library of Congress Cataloging-in-Publication Data:
eISBN: 978-3-95-830983-8; Print ISBN: 978-0-9975371-8-5
Tennin, Kyla Latrice.
All Natural Soups & Stews
Pages cm; copyrighted materials.
    1.   Health-Nutrition-Diet-Fitness. 2. Cooking. 3. Fitness.
Library of Congress Catalog Card Number: 2016907241

Print Book Edition, License Note

This book is licensed for your personal enjoyment only. This book may not be re-sold or given away to other people. If you would like to share this book with another person, please purchase an additional copy for each recipient. If you're reading this book and did not purchase it, or it was not purchased for your use only, then please return to your favorite book retailer and purchase your own copy. Thank you for respecting the hard work of this author.

Also Note

In this book, Ms. Latrice begins by explaining a *fast* that she has created, tested and tried, which contributed to her weight loss, weight management and healthy eating lifestyle journey. She has also written this book due to there being so many books, health, weight-loss and "diet" programs currently on the global market. The programs and books she has seen and reviewed are too long, too thick, have too much information and many times, are difficult for people to read. This book was written to *simplify and shorten* how to lose weight and maintain your health, for life. It is based on personal experience and is still done today. It's an effective solution.

"All Natural Soups & Stews"

Table of Contents

DEDICATION

This cookbook is dedicated to men and women around the world that have dealt with or are beginning to deal with food addiction, obesity and/or declining health.

I also dedicate this book to those whom have been "Mirage's" in life; overlooked, betrayed, not good enough, slandered, mistreated, misunderstood, misrepresented and even treated unfairly because of their weight or how they looked on the **outside** to others, when in fact, on the **inside** there's greater.

This new cookbook is also dedicated to men and women around the world that want to
shift from being ordinary to extraordinary and accomplishing what others said you would never be able to do again or never be able to do at all.

Here's to the New You!

ACKNOWLEDGMENTS

I want to *say thank you* to anyone whom has ever betrayed,
rejected, mistreated, teased, and misused
or looked down upon me. You helped me become GREATER
and launched me into my destiny.

Whenever someone throws bricks at you, use them to *"build"*.
Build something greater; even your mansion.

And whenever you face opposition, "know" that it is actually
an opportunity; a set-back for a set-up to secure the victory,
rejection for rewards, pain for gain, lack for prosperity to
leave a legacy, misery for miracles and put downs for
promotion.

IT'S YOUR TIME...*to bounce back!*

Let's Get Healthy!

AUTHOR'S NOTE

All Natural Soups & Stews
Copyright © 2014
Ms. Kyla Latrice, Inc.
All Rights Reserved.

AFFIDAVIT

All content written herein is of opinion, from personal experience and of suggestion. Individual slow-cooker recipes (for weight loss or weight management) and new eating plan results may vary from person to person and no results are guaranteed.

You must put forth effort and do the work necessary to take charge of changing your life and *losing weight*. I did and so can you.

You can also utilize this cookbook if you have already met your weight loss goals and just want to stay healthy with recipes that will keep your metabolism in check and body running smoothly.

Be sure to wash all fruits, vegetables, foods, etc. thoroughly before beginning any new
eating or meal plan.

ALL RIGHTS RESERVED

No portion of this publication may be reproduced, stored in any electronic system, or transmitted in any form by any means; electronic, mechanical,
photocopy, recording or otherwise, without written permission from the author.
Brief quotations may be used in literary reviews with the consent of the author and publisher.

"ON-THE-GO"

This cookbook *(and all of my cookbooks,*
books, workbook and manuals) can be read and applied in
airports, on trains, at work on your lunch break,
in grocery stores while shopping for and planning your
weekly meals, at bookstore cafes,
at restaurants *(for quick decision making; to remember your*
health and/or weight loss goals) and even in shopping malls.

In addition, *this book can be brought to*
fast food restaurants (to pull up and look through to remember
your goals before ordering), at the park (before a jog or
potluck), during your hotel stays,
on vacations and at airport food counters when ordering your
meals and drinks *(so you remember your goals and what to*
eat and drink).

This cookbook has been made available
on mobile devices via Adobe Digital Editions and DRM
(Digital Rights Management).

WORLD STATISTICS

Obesity and Childhood Obesity
Centers for Disease Control and Prevention
http://www.cdc.gov/obesity/data/adult.html
http://www.cdc.gov/nchs/fastats/obesity-overweight.htm

Harvard School of Public Health
http://www.hsph.harvard.edu/obesity-prevention-
source/obesity-trends/

World Health Organization
http://www.who.int/topics/obesity/en/

Stroke Awareness and Prevention
http://www.cdc.gov/stroke/facts.htm

Diabetes Awareness and Prevention
Centers for Disease Control and Prevention
http://www.cdc.gov/diabetes/data/statistics/2014statisticsrepor
t.html

American Diabetes Association
http://www.diabetes.org/diabetes-basics/statistics/

ALL NATURAL SOUPS & STEWS

"FASTING"

WHAT IS FASTING?

➤ Fasting is abstaining from PLEASURABLE foods for a certain amount of time to FOCUS on things that are more important than pleasurable foods to get to the root of what is causing your poor health, obesity, relationships and quality of life.

➤ It is not a hunger strike.

➤ You're able to see into your life better and rid it of the bad when you pull away from portion after portion at the dinner table, lunch buffet after buffet with friends and co-workers, nightly binge eating and drinking (whether alcohol, sodas, sugary drinks and the like) and dessert or movie nights on the sofa with a large pizza box and donuts.

➤ Fasting helps you pinpoint where you overdo things (overindulge), gets you back on track and teaches you how to eat, "in moderation" (balance), for your health and for a better life.

➤ Your body may not like eating healthy for the first few days (especially if you have never fasted before), but it will adjust.

REASONS FOR FASTING:

➤ It produces a physical discipline (especially for how, when, where and *what* you eat).

➤ It rids the body of toxins (just like exercise does when you sweat); cleansing your body and digestive tracts, improving your health and weight.

Note: If you are on medication, consult your physician before any *fast*.

BENEFITS OF FASTING:

➢ It strengthens *you* and your body.

➢ Fasting brings joy, happiness and *energy* to your life; and fruits, vegetables, oils, etc. are quite inexpensive. Make a list and shop for your ingredients before you begin.

➢ You become very aware of *what* and *how much* you eat. You also begin to pay more attention to when and where you always eat/drink and what leads you to OVEREATING.

➢ Fasting brings humility, revelation and an overall healthy lifestyle (mind, emotions, intellect, etc.).

TYPICAL TYPES OF FASTS:

Sometimes people fast the following from their lives:

➢ Television (even the internet, social media or video games) for one day, three days or even one week, television during certain hours of the day (to break a cycle of watching certain shows they may be addicted to (like food) that aren't good for them.

....or

➢ To break a cycle of "certain foods" they may eat while watching certain television shows.

➢ Fasting to abstain from all pleasurable foods and red meats, eating only fruits, vegetables, clear soups, cereals (no white sugar), water, diluted fruit juices (100% juices only) and/or grains.

➢ Some people even fast people (bad acquaintances, friendships or relationships), leading eventually to moving away from those person's completely, for a better life and health. Your health is your life.

➢ Many people fast for 24 hours, three days, seven days, 14 days, 21 days or longer. My success and learning my body as well as other persons bodies (whom have fasted when I have fasted) has come from "closely monitoring" how the body reacts to each of these fasts (particularly "21 days") and I've noticed some things and have sculpted recipes to help others find that tremendous success in many areas of their lives as well.

➢ Fasts should always be broken slowly, especially if you have been on an "extended fast" (a fast for more than 30 days, a salad only fast, a smoothie only fast or even a clear soup only fast).

➢ Gradually get back into "regular food", until you can completely commit to "healthy food" (and a regular healthy lifestyle); such as having juices for a couple of days, then fruits, vegetables, grains and adding meats back into your diet last, if applicable.

➢ Typically, people have six meals per day (three main meals (breakfast, lunch and dinner) and three snacks). For each of my Fasts or Recipes, you determine how many meals. Don't worry, fruits and vegetables do not cause obesity, they prevent it. Yet, always watch your portion sizes, in general, and with soups, stews and anything that has meat included. Never eat meat in excess.

➢ You can even choose to eat one meal per day for 21 days (there are enough recipes listed in this book), a snack, have 5-8 bottles of water and be sure to get a nap in and some exercise during the week. As you advance you can mix your salad fast with a smoothie fast and detox fast by doing one of the fasts, each per week, for 21 days, etc.

THE *"SALAD FAST"*
BIRTH

Kyla Latrice is a native of Marks, MS and enjoys food and traveling. Being from a small town and a country gal, she set her goals high. Graduating from a private institution with a Bachelor of Arts Degree (BA) *(women's studies and health background; pre-medicine)* and a Master's Degree (MBA) in Business Administration with **Executive Education at Harvard and Stanford** along with several certifications and nearly 50-80 self-study coursework in legal, intellectual property and self-help, she has become one of the leading entrepreneurs of her time.

Currently Ms. Latrice is finishing up her Doctoral Honorary Degree *(Doctor of Management in Organizational Leadership)* and continues to serve on Board of Directors throughout the world for various causes; still relating to her life's purpose and corporations work. Ms. Latrice travels extensively for speaking engagements in the areas of health, wellness, obesity, poverty, domestic violence, branding, image, leadership, mentoring, business, entrepreneurship and the like.

To date, Ms. Latrice has mentored with over 20 plus organizations *(from elementary to senior citizen)*, helping others overcome issues she has faced.

With her first *corporate* job opportunity being at a "Health Food Restaurant" *(when she was age 15 or 16)* to work as a deli attendant at the deli bar, hostess *(when others were out for the day)* and bakery attendant as well as a chef in the *salad bar*.

Her main role was to attend to the deli, to prepare healthy pasta salads, healthy sandwiches, healthy shakes, healthy sundaes and *healthy smoothies*. However, Ms. Latrice was blessed with the opportunity to be called upon whenever management needed her help in the other areas as well, **to continue learning**. This gave Ms. Latrice very valuable experience and a "look" into health and business ownership, a bit deeper, which still remains with her today.

THE *"SALAD FAST"* BIRTH

KYLA LATRICE
BEFORE
21 DAY SALAD FASTS

Ms. Latrice's *(on the left in the photo)* Corporations are inclusive of health restaurants, retail stores, property and land as well as product development organizations along with nonprofit foundations to care for the displaced, homeless.

Further, Ms. Latrice's love for food turned into obesity when her life took a turn in the early 2000's during domestic violence, sinful relationships, bad friendships, emotional binge eating and more; then again in the 2000's with another domestic violence relationship, obesity slander from family members, mental and spiritual abuse, abortion, home foreclosure, vehicle repossession and much *more*, which all have an effect on health, but she made sure her Corporations still stood; to help others.

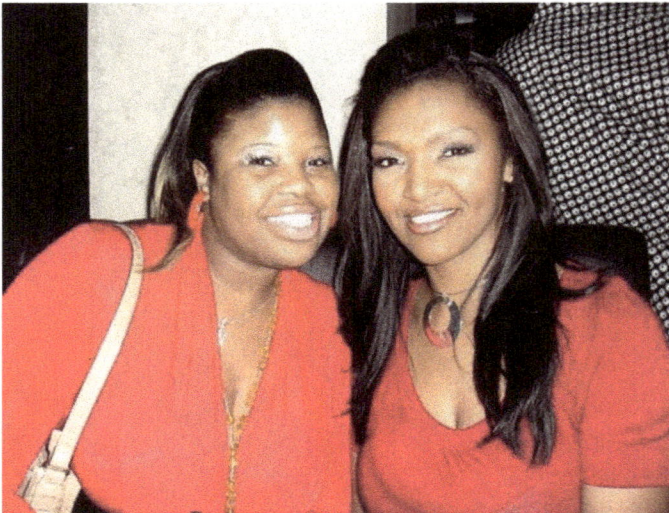

THE *"SALAD FAST"*
BIRTH

KYLA LATRICE
"IN THE MIDDLE"
AFTER GAINING WEIGHT BACK FOR
A SECOND TIME
21 DAY SALAD FASTS

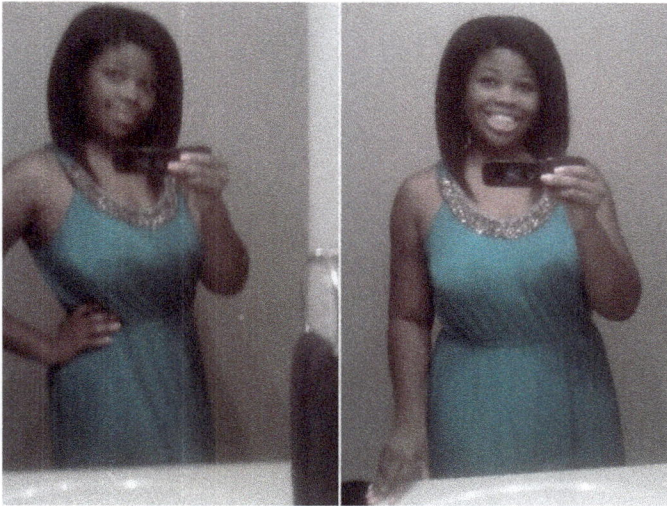

THE *"SALAD FAST"* BIRTH

KYLA LATRICE
AFTER
21 DAY SALAD FASTS

THE FINALE

ALL NATURAL SOUPS & STEWS

Many factors can contribute to obesity, such as abuse *(mental, spiritual, physical, sexual)*, poor eating habits, environment, bad friendships, sin and more. Personally, I, myself, was never taught how to eat, I did not know what to eat *(that was truly healthy for me)* and I did not know how to deal with life's problems.

Nevertheless, how can someone teach you what they don't know? My first encounter with obesity was when I was a model and went from a size 0 to a size 20/22, **weighing close to 300 pounds** *(then I lost nearly 115 pounds after prayer and seeking a remedy)*.

The second encounter was when I gained some of the first encounters weight back and went from a size 14/16 to a size 4/6 and fitting a 7/8 in jeans, losing 68 pounds. Today, I am going to share my secrets to success with you *(the birth of the "21 Day Salad Fast")* and how I made it out over the years ***and*** kept the weight off. Let's get started and healthy, for life!

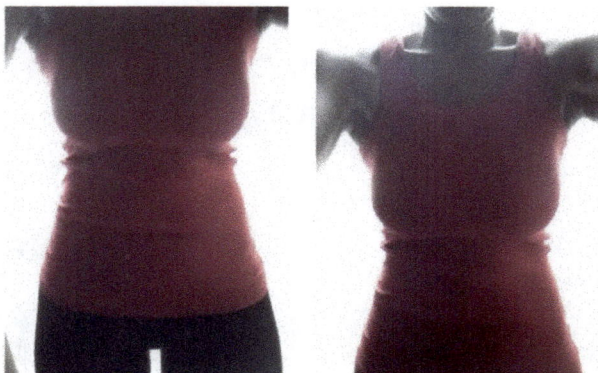

GETTING HEALTHY
LIFESTYLE CHANGE

ALL NATURAL SOUPS & STEWS

Prepare to lose weight on the "Salad Fast" (this is not a "diet", this is an "eating plan" to reprogram your mind, body and metabolism about how to eat (portion control) and regarding what foods you should and should not be eating). It is designed to help you become healthier. Before starting this fast and any of my eating *plans ("The 21 Day Smoothie Fast" and "The 21 Day Salad Fast" as well as "All Natural Soups and Stews")*, allow yourself "one week" to prepare for the fast and eating plan by removing the following from your life:

➤ Negative relationships and friendships; they block you from doing well in life and succeeding, when people begin to see you doing well, they tend to not like it. Choose friendships and associations wisely. Be creative.

➤ Bad acquaintances; they will eventually want what you have and will cause betrayal to take place in your life through a "set-up" to sabotage all of your hard work. Always keep moving forward.

➤ Remove the following (slowly) from your daily meals (eating habits) because they contribute to weight gain (some quicker than others): soda, breads, pastas, candy bars and the like and eating second, third and fourth portions of your food. You only need one portion. Don't eat the rest!

➤ Replace all sodas with diet soda until you can cut soda out of your daily meal plan completely; only drink soda if absolutely necessary *(a lemon-lime beverage)* because there is nothing else to drink. For example, while traveling.

➤ Remove all "junk food" (cakes, pies, chips, all kinds of desserts and the like) from your kitchen.

➢ For breads, certain kinds make the weight gain skyrocket; be careful about pizza. Pasta should be limited just like soda, having it only if absolutely necessary, but once every 2-4 months is okay, just like donuts, to stay **balanced** and give your body a break from always eating healthy.

➢ Again, you only need one portion of food, per meal, work on this and you'll see results quicker.

➢ Increase your water intake to 5-8 bottled waters a day; bring a bottle with you everywhere you go so you'll be forced to drink it *(instead of something else)* and will program your body to like it *(whether you like it frozen, warm or cold)*.

➢ When you're out to eating with others, begin selecting items from menus that help *(not hinder)* your **new eating plan**, for example, order a "grilled chicken wrap with a side salad and small water" instead of a double cheeseburger, french fries and large soda. Never super-size, it wastes your results and time spent on improving your health.

➢ If you have not already, purchase my books: *"The 21 Day Smoothie Fast"* and *"The 21 Day Salad Fast"* to begin, to continue your weight loss and new you.

➢ And again, remember, commit to single portion eating, eating smaller portions (always have more vegetables on your plate than poultry/ meat), and increase your water intake *(remember to use the restroom)*. Let's begin.

GETTING HEALTHY
SET GOALS

Feel free to purchase my "A New Healthy You Workout Workbook" *(to go with your **new eating plan** and my "fasts" cookbooks* or a composition notebook from any retailer to make your own journal to measure the following (even if you need to do so at your primary care physician's office, a free clinic or go to a free health assessment machine in a retail store location that has one):

Record a written record of each:

> ➢ Your Cholesterol Level.
> ➢ Blood Pressure and Vision Check.
> ➢ Your actual Height Weight, Height, Bust/Chest and Hips size (write down your goals of where you want to be in the next week, three months, six months and year).
> ➢ Record your weight, chest/bust, hips and waist size every Saturday morning at 7am.
> ➢ Stroll through a department store and notate clothing (or take a camera phone photo) you plan on fitting into someday and notate your current sizes and then return in three months to see how you're fairing up towards your goals.
> ➢ Pick up my *"A New Healthy You Workout Workbook"* or list in your journal, your reasons for losing weight, changing your life and changing your eating habits.

> ➤ Your BMI (Body Mass Index) and where you are versus where you're supposed to be for your height, weight, age and gender.
> ➤ Bottles of "cold water" listed in most of my books recipes sections are in reference to drinking 4-5 bottles of 16 fl oz bottles of water, which is equivalent to 8-10 glasses of water per day.
> ➤ Water is vital for living and for being healthy.
> ➤ The amount of water within the human body is typically 50-65% water and in infants, 78%.
> ➤ Water assists your body with digesting food and getting nutrients from the foods you have eaten to your blood, brain and other parts of your body, in order to function; emptying the body of waste and toxins, helps deliver oxygen to the body, helps prevent constipation and even regulates body temperature (in your cells, organs and tissues).

A (BMI) Chart is below for your convenience.

BMI	<(less than) 18.5	=	Underweight
BMI	18.5-24.9	=	Normal Weight
BMI	25-29.9	=	Overweight
BMI	>(more than) 30	=	Obese

GETTING HEALTHY
WHILE TRAVELING

If you'll be traveling by airplane, helicopter or private jet (smile):

 ➢ Research where you will be eating ahead of time (food choices, ingredients and prices).
 ➢ Bring bottled water.
 ➢ Resist vending machines and relying of fast food at your final destination.
 ➢ Bring your own snacks (trail mix, cashews, a banana, apple slices, peanuts) and
 ➢ Workout for free in your hotel room, taking the stairs instead of elevators and walking at the Mall.

If traveling by car:

 ➢ Pack your own cooler with ice for your bottled waters, fruits and raw vegetables.
 ➢ Consider bringing a bag of oranges & any other food that can be eaten warm or cold on the road.

If you'll be traveling by bus, train, or other means:

 ➢ Research where you will be eating ahead of time (food choices, ingredients and prices).
 ➢ Bring bottled water.
 ➢ Bring your own snacks (trail mix, cashews, a banana, apple slices, peanuts for the long trip) and
 ➢ Bring something to read or play, to keep your mind off of food and *fictious* hunger.
 ➢ At your destination, stand more than you sit (to keep your body moving) and since you have been sitting during traveling for your trip.

SPINACH

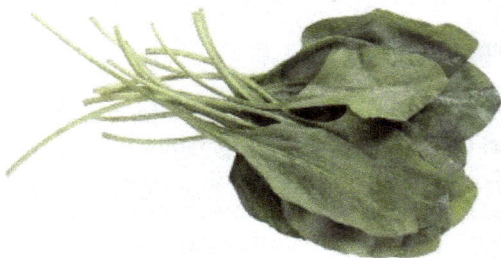

Photo Credit: Smarnad
Freedigitalphotos.net

ALL NATURAL SOUPS & STEWS

GETTING HEALTHY
YOUR NEW WORKOUT PLAN

During my both times of being obese, I never worked out at a gym nor went outside of my home to run *(weighing in at 278 pounds and trying to start my "new me" as a jogger was terrible on my knees)* to lose weight, I did it all at home, on the floor, in a compact room, near a closet. I suggest you begin a "workout regime" by doing simple workouts, such as crunches, stretching, leg lifts and a few push-ups.

Everyone cannot do cardio in the gym (paid membership prices or because of lack of transportation), running outside or bouncing around in-doors for 1-3 hours like actors and actresses on television, whom are likely being *paid monetary* compensation or by other means to film the infomercial.

Remain constant and do this 3-4 times a week, for 15-35 minutes each day. On your workout OFF days, do 100 crunches before going to bed. Consider purchasing my "Workout Workbook" to keep up with your Fitness Plan. In addition, you burn calories when you sleep, by drinking water, by exercising (which helps you live longer as well) and by **movement** (whether your arms, legs, looking out of a window, etc.).

Furthermore, water helps break down food and helps food digest. Your can also do a "mental workout" by cutting out negative people, places and things from your life.

You'll find that you have more peace in your brain and life, when you replace them with reading inspirational books, movies, community work and exercise or things you love, such as knitting, a ball game, taking a site seeing road trip (alone) every now and then or mentoring someone.

Notes

_____

_____

_____

_____

_____

_____

_____

_____

_____

_____

_____

_____

_____

_____

_____

_____

_____

_____

_____

_____

_____

_____

_____

_____

_____

_____

_____

_____

THE SIX MONTH RULE
GIVE IT *"TIME"*

THE SIX-MONTH RULE
On a 21-Day Salad Fast, weight [pounds] have been known to drop quickly for many people. However, the goal here is to also keep the weight off. Stay focused and be committed to at least six-months of "health work".

Remember to journal your progress.

There's something about when you write things down, they get *ACCOMPLISHED!* Also give yourself a total of six-months to work on your "New You" simply because you may lose inches first and not weight, until your weight catches up with your inches (this is what took place with me; loosing 10-12 pounds per month).

Inches first then one day the weight just fell off. And for others, sometimes weight first, then inches.

GO BACK TO THE DEPARTMENT STORE
Revisit those same department stores that you went to on the first week of your new lifestyle change, try on new clothing sizes to see where you are with your goals.

I suggest that you "mentally shop" for a new suit, a dinner dress, clothing for you next vacation (Hawaii maybe), your first pair of skinny jeans or baseball gear to wear to a game; all after you have reached your goals; to *CELEBRATE!*

Boiler Pots, Crock-Pots and Hand Blenders (for purees)
Examples & where to purchase:

AMAZON.COM
www.sears.com and www.gandermountain.com
(King Kooker Boiler Pot with Steamed Rim)
http://www.iheartthemart.com/82901/
(Triple, Small Crock-Pots)
http://www.walmart.com/ip/Curtis-Stone-Hardstuff-Saucepan-with-Lid/39943029 (Curtis Stone Saucepan w/Lid)
http://www.amazon.com/Brinkmann-812-9160-S-60-Quart-Boiling-Basket/dp/B0044SZLJ4 (24 Qrt or do 60Qrt if you have a family; Brinkmann Boiler Pot, Lower Priced)

www.amazon.com (Bayou Classic 8000 Boiler Pots, as well as Stainless Steel)
www.OverStock.com and www.macys.com
(Hamilton Beach Electric Hand Blender and Cuisinart Hand Blender)

FOOD SERVICE WAREHOUSE
www.foodservicewarehouse.com

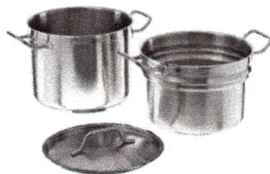

Photo Credit: UpdateInternational the Brand and Cuisinart

"SOUPS & STEWS"
RECIPES

Sometimes you need to give your *body* a rest from what you have been eating regularly, *such as meats*, especially those that take quite a bit of time to digest and to rid the body of toxins that came in through certain foods eaten.

Here are some of my favorite natural soups and stews recipes that I have created to help you get the food rest you need, whether for a day, week or even month; to enjoy other foods and ways of cooking. Variety in life is good.

For Cooking, you can either utilize a slow-cooker, crock-pot or a boiler on the stove. Within this book, to make sure everyone has the utensils needed, you can simply use a boiler pot on a traditional stove (whether electric or gas; gas cooks food more evenly and thoroughly). Enjoy!

GOOD OLD-FASHIONED
VEGETABLE SOUP

DAY 1
(GOOD OLD-FASHIONED VEGETARIAN SOUP)

Typically makes 4-6 servings and lasts a few days, but utilize a "Small" Boiler Pot or "Small Sized Crock-Pot" (for best results) for smaller portions to watch your weight, prevent over-eating and watch your sodium (salt) intake.

Main Ingredients:
Into a Small Boiler Pot
Certified 100% Organic (home grown is best) Vegetables

Add 1 cup of diced onion, Add 1 cup of diced green bell pepper, Add 1 cup of diced red bell pepper, Add 1 cup of corn, Add 1 cup of diced parsley, Add 1 cup of diced roma tomatoes (both yellow and red), Add 1 cup of diced celery, Add a dash of salt, Add 1/2 teaspoon of ground red pepper, Add a dash of pepper, Add 1 diced garlic clove, Add 1/2 teaspoon of thyme, Add 2 teaspoons of certified 100% organic extra-virgin olive oil, Add 4-5 cups of (purified) water (regular cold tap water is fine as well), Bring to a boil

Cook for a few hours
Cook until thoroughly heated and boiled
Serve immediately, after cooling (5-10 minutes)

Additional Notes: if desired:
Add 1 cup of any (diced) 100% certified organic, farm raised, grass fed "baked" lemon-pepper and Greek seasoned meat

SWEET POTATO STEW

DAY 2
(SWEET POTATO STEW)

Typically makes 4-6 servings and lasts a few days, but utilize a "Small" Boiler Pot or "Small Sized Crock-Pot" (for best results) for smaller portions to watch your weight, prevent over-eating and watch your sodium (salt) intake.

Main Ingredients:
Into a Small Boiler Pot
Add 3-4 diced (into small squares) sweet potatoes

Add 1 cup of diced onion, Add 1 cup of diced green bell pepper, Add 1 cup of diced red bell pepper, Add 1 cup of corn, Add 1 cup of diced parsley, Add 1 cup of diced roma tomatoes (both yellow and red), Add 1 cup of diced celery, Add a dash of salt, Add 1/2 teaspoon of ground red pepper, Add a dash of pepper, Add 1 diced garlic clove, Add 1/2 teaspoon of thyme, Add 2 teaspoons of certified 100% organic extra-virgin olive oil, Add 4-5 cups of (purified) water (regular cold tap water is fine as well), Bring to a boil

Cook for a few hours
Cook until thoroughly heated and boiled
After cooling (20 minutes), puree the stew with a hand blender
Heat again for another 35 minutes until brought to a simmer
Serve immediately, after cooling (5-10 minutes)

Additional Notes: if desired:
Add 1 cup of any (diced) 100% certified organic, farm raised, grass fed "baked" lemon-pepper and Greek seasoned meat

CABBAGE & BARLEY SOUP

DAY 3
(CABBAGE & BARLEY SOUP)

Typically makes 4-6 servings and lasts a few days, but utilize a "Small" Boiler Pot or "Small Sized Crock-Pot" (for best results) for smaller portions to watch your weight, prevent over-eating and watch your sodium (salt) intake.

Main Ingredients:
Into a Small Boiler Pot
Add a cabbage halved and 1-2 cups of organic barley

Add 1 cup of diced onion, Add 1 cup of diced green bell pepper, Add 1 cup of diced red bell pepper, Add 1 cup of corn, Add 1 cup of diced parsley, Add 1 cup of diced roma tomatoes (both yellow and red), Add 1 cup of diced celery, Add a dash of salt, Add 1/2 teaspoon of ground red pepper, Add a dash of pepper, Add 1 diced garlic clove, Add 1/2 teaspoon of thyme, Add 2 teaspoons of certified 100% organic extra-virgin olive oil, Add 4-5 cups of (purified) water (regular cold tap water is fine as well), Bring to a boil

Cook for a few hours
Cook until thoroughly heated and boiled
Serve immediately, after cooling (5-10 minutes)

Additional Notes: if desired:
Add 1 cup of any (diced) 100% certified organic, farm raised, grass fed "baked" lemon-pepper and Greek seasoned meat

BUTTERNUT SQUASH STEW

DAY 4
(BUTTERNUT SQUASH STEW)

Typically makes 4-6 servings and lasts a few days, but utilize a "Small" Boiler Pot or "Small Sized Crock-Pot" (for best results) for smaller portions to watch your weight, prevent over-eating and watch your sodium (salt) intake.

Main Ingredients:
Into a Small Boiler Pot
Add 3-4 diced (into small squares) butternut squash

Add 1 cup of diced onion, Add 1 cup of diced green bell pepper, Add 1 cup of diced red bell pepper, Add 1 cup of corn, Add 1 cup of diced parsley, Add 1 cup of diced roma tomatoes (both yellow and red), Add 1 cup of diced celery, Add a dash of salt, Add 1/2 teaspoon of ground red pepper, Add a dash of pepper, Add 1 diced garlic clove, Add 1/2 teaspoon of thyme, Add 2 teaspoons of certified 100% organic extra-virgin olive oil, Add 4-5 cups of (purified) water (regular cold tap water is fine as well), Bring to a boil

Cook for a few hours
Cook until thoroughly heated and boiled
After cooling (20 minutes), puree the stew with a hand blender
Heat again for another 35 minutes until brought to a simmer
Serve immediately, after cooling (5-10 minutes)

Additional Notes: if desired:
Add 1 cup of any (diced) 100% certified organic, farm raised, grass fed "baked" lemon-pepper and Greek seasoned meat

TOMATO BASIL SOUP

DAY 5
(TOMATO BASIL SOUP)

Typically makes 4-6 servings and lasts a few days, but utilize a "Small" Boiler Pot or "Small Sized Crock-Pot" (for best results) for smaller portions to watch your weight, prevent over-eating and watch your sodium (salt) intake.

Main Ingredients:
Into a Small Boiler Pot
Add 4-6 diced (into small squares) large organic tomatoes and 2-3 tablespoons of organic basil

Add 1 cup of diced onion, Add 1 cup of diced green bell pepper, Add 1 cup of diced red bell pepper, Add 1 cup of corn, Add 1 cup of diced parsley, Add 1 cup of diced roma tomatoes (both yellow and red), Smoked Paprika, Add 1 cup of diced celery, Add a dash of salt, Add 1/2 teaspoon of ground red pepper, Add a dash of pepper, Add 1 diced garlic clove, Add ½ cup of chopped parsley, Add 2 teaspoons of certified 100% organic extra-virgin olive oil, Add 4-5 cups of (purified) water (regular cold tap water is fine as well), Bring to a boil

Cook for a few hours
Cook until thoroughly heated and boiled
Serve immediately, after cooling (5-10 minutes)

Additional Notes: if desired:
Add 1 cup of any (diced) 100% certified organic, farm raised, grass fed "baked" lemon-pepper and Greek seasoned meat

GOOD OLD-FASHIONED MINESTRONE STEW

DAY 6
(GOOD OLD-FASHIONED MINESTRONE STEW)

Typically makes 4-6 servings and lasts a few days, but utilize a "Small" Boiler Pot or "Small Sized Crock-Pot" (for best results) for smaller portions to watch your weight, prevent over-eating and watch your sodium (salt) intake.

Main Ingredients:
Into a Small Boiler Pot
Add 3-4 diced (into small squares) sweet potatoes

Add 1 cup of diced onion, Add 1 cup of diced green bell pepper, Add 1 cup of diced red bell pepper, Add 1 cup of corn, Add 1 cup of diced parsley, Add 1 cup of carrots, 1 can of rinsed kidney beans, 1 cup of green beans, 1 tablespoon of dried oregano, 1 cup of whole wheat elbow pasta, Add 1 cup of diced celery, Add a dash of salt, Add 1/2 teaspoon of ground red pepper, Add a dash of pepper, Add 1 diced garlic clove, Add 1/2 teaspoon of thyme, Add 2 teaspoons of certified 100% organic extra-virgin olive oil, Add 4-5 cups of (purified) water (regular cold tap water is fine as well)
Bring to a boil

Cook for a few hours
Cook until thoroughly heated and boiled
After cooling (20 minutes), puree the stew with a hand blender
Heat again for another 35 minutes until brought to a simmer
Serve immediately, after cooling (5-10 minutes)

Additional Notes: if desired:
Add 1 cup of any (diced) 100% certified organic, farm raised, grass fed "baked" lemon-pepper and Greek seasoned meat

BROCCOLI SOUP

DAY 7
(BROCCOLI SOUP)

Typically makes 4-6 servings and lasts a few days, but utilize a "Small" Boiler Pot or "Small Sized Crock-Pot" (for best results) for smaller portions to watch your weight, prevent over-eating and watch your sodium (salt) intake.

Main Ingredients:
Into a Small Boiler Pot
Add one full pot of organic (washed & rinsed) broccoli (cut into florets)

Add 1 cup of diced onion, Add 1 cup of diced green bell pepper, Add 1 cup of diced red bell pepper, Add 1 cup of corn, Add 1 cup of diced parsley, Add 1 cup of diced roma tomatoes (both yellow and red), Add 1 cup of diced celery, Add a dash of salt, Add 1/2 teaspoon of ground red pepper, Add a dash of pepper, Add 1 diced garlic clove, Add 1/2 teaspoon of thyme, Add 2 teaspoons of certified 100% organic extra-virgin olive oil, Add 4-5 cups of (purified) water (regular cold tap water is fine as well), Bring to a boil

Cook for a few hours
Cook until thoroughly heated and boiled
Serve immediately, after cooling (5-10 minutes)

Additional Notes: if desired:
Add 1 cup of any (diced) 100% certified organic, farm raised, grass fed "baked" lemon-pepper and Greek seasoned meat

CAULIFLOWER STEW

DAY 8
(CAULIFLOWER STEW)

Typically makes 4-6 servings and lasts a few days, but utilize a "Small" Boiler Pot or "Small Sized Crock-Pot" (for best results) for smaller portions to watch your weight, prevent over-eating and watch your sodium (salt) intake.

Main Ingredients:
Into a Small Boiler Pot
Add one full pot of organic (washed & rinsed) cauliflower (use white or purple), cut into florets

Add 1 cup of diced onion, Add 1 cup of diced green bell pepper, Add 1 cup of diced red bell pepper, Add 1 cup of corn, Add 1 cup of diced parsley, Add 1 cup of diced roma tomatoes (both yellow and red), Add 1 cup of diced celery, Add a dash of salt, Add 1/2 teaspoon of ground red pepper, Add a dash of pepper, Add 1 diced garlic clove, Add 1/2 teaspoon of thyme, Add 2 teaspoons of certified 100% organic extra-virgin olive oil, Add 4-5 cups of (purified) water (regular cold tap water is fine as well), Bring to a boil

Cook for a few hours
Cook until thoroughly heated and boiled
After cooling (20 minutes), puree the stew with a hand blender
Heat again for another 35 minutes until brought to a simmer
Serve immediately, after cooling (5-10 minutes)

Additional Notes: if desired:
Add 1 cup of any (diced) 100% certified organic, farm raised, grass fed "baked" lemon-pepper and Greek seasoned meat

RADISHES AND
GREEN-ONION SOUP

DAY 9
(RADISHES AND GREEN-ONION SOUP)

Typically makes 4-6 servings and lasts a few days, but utilize a "Small" Boiler Pot or "Small Sized Crock-Pot" (for best results) for smaller portions to watch your weight, prevent over-eating and watch your sodium (salt) intake.

Main Ingredients:
Into a Small Boiler Pot
Add 4-6 diced (into small squares) radishes and 2-3 cups of finely diced green onion or scallions

Add 1 cup of diced onion, Add 1 cup of diced green bell pepper, Add 1 cup of diced red bell pepper, Add 1 cup of corn, Add 1 cup of diced parsley, Add 1 cup of diced roma tomatoes (both yellow and red), Add 1 cup of diced celery, Add a dash of salt, Add 1/2 teaspoon of ground red pepper, Add a dash of pepper, Add 1 diced garlic clove, Add 1/2 teaspoon of thyme, Add 2 teaspoons of certified 100% organic extra-virgin olive oil, Add 4-5 cups of (purified) water (regular cold tap water is fine as well), Bring to a boil

Cook for a few hours
Cook until thoroughly heated and boiled
Serve immediately, after cooling (5-10 minutes)

Additional Notes: if desired:
Add 1 cup of any (diced) 100% certified organic, farm raised, grass fed "baked" lemon-pepper and Greek seasoned meat

ZUCCHINI &
RED PEPPER STEW

DAY 10
(ZUCCHINI & RED PEPPER STEW)

Typically makes 4-6 servings and lasts a few days, but utilize a "Small" Boiler Pot or "Small Sized Crock-Pot" (for best results) for smaller portions to watch your weight, prevent over-eating and watch your sodium (salt) intake.

Main Ingredients:
Into a Small Boiler Pot
Add 3-4 diced (into small squares) Zucchini (yellow or green), 2-3 finely diced red peppers (bell)

Add 1 cup of diced onion, Add 1 cup of diced green bell pepper, Add 1 cup of diced red bell pepper, Add 1 cup of corn, Add 1 cup of diced parsley, Add 1 cup of diced roma tomatoes (both yellow and red), Add 1 cup of diced celery, Add a dash of salt, Add 1/2 teaspoon of ground red pepper, Add a dash of pepper, Add 1 diced garlic clove, Add 1/2 teaspoon of thyme, Add 2 teaspoons of certified 100% organic extra-virgin olive oil, Add 4-5 cups of (purified) water (regular cold tap water is fine as well), Bring to a boil

Cook for a few hours
Cook until thoroughly heated and boiled
After cooling (20 minutes), puree the stew with a hand blender
Heat again for another 35 minutes until brought to a simmer
Serve immediately, after cooling (5-10 minutes)

Additional Notes: if desired:
Add 1 cup of any (diced) 100% certified organic, farm raised, grass fed "baked" lemon-pepper and Greek seasoned meat

SPINACH & WILD
MUSHROOMS SOUP

DAY 11
(SPINACH & WILD MUSHROOMS SOUP)

Typically makes 4-6 servings and lasts a few days, but utilize a "Small" Boiler Pot or "Small Sized Crock-Pot" (for best results) for smaller portions to watch your weight, prevent over-eating and watch your sodium (salt) intake.

Main Ingredients:
Into a Small Boiler Pot
Add 3-4 cups of diced spinach stalks and 2-3 cups of chopped organic wild mushrooms (any kind)

Add 1 cup of diced onion, Add 1 cup of diced green bell pepper, Add 1 cup of diced red bell pepper, Add 1 cup of corn, Add 1 cup of diced parsley, Add 1 cup of diced roma tomatoes (both yellow and red), Add 1 cup of diced celery, Add a dash of salt, Add 1/2 teaspoon of ground red pepper, Add a dash of pepper, Add 1 diced garlic clove, Add 1/2 teaspoon of thyme, Add 2 teaspoons of certified 100% organic extra-virgin olive oil, Add 4-5 cups of (purified) water (regular cold tap water is fine as well), Bring to a boil

Cook for a few hours
Cook until thoroughly heated and boiled
Serve immediately, after cooling (5-10 minutes)

Additional Notes: **if desired:**
Add 1 cup of any (diced) 100% certified organic, farm raised, grass fed "baked" lemon-pepper and Greek seasoned meat

BEAN & WHOLE WHEAT TORTILLA STEW

ALL NATURAL SOUPS & STEWS

DAY 12
(BEAN & WHOLE WHEAT TORTILLA STEW)

Typically makes 4-6 servings and lasts a few days, but utilize a "Small" Boiler Pot or "Small Sized Crock-Pot" (for best results) for smaller portions to watch your weight, prevent over-eating and watch your sodium (salt) intake.

Main Ingredients:
Into a Small Boiler Pot
Add 3-4 cups of whole wheat tortillas chips/sticks (as a garnish at the end) and 2 cans of low-sodium red beans

Add 1 cup of diced onion, Add 1 cup of diced green bell pepper, Add 1 cup of diced red bell pepper, Add 1 cup of corn, Add 1 cup of diced parsley, Add 1 cup of diced roma tomatoes (both yellow and red), Add 1 cup of diced celery, Add a dash of salt, Add 1/2 teaspoon of ground red pepper, Add a dash of pepper, Add 1 diced garlic clove, Add 1/2 teaspoon of thyme, Add 2 teaspoons of certified 100% organic extra-virgin olive oil, Add 4-5 cups of (purified) water (regular cold tap water is fine as well), Bring to a boil

Cook for a few hours
Cook until thoroughly heated and boiled
Serve immediately, after cooling (5-10 minutes)
After cooling (20 minutes), puree the stew with a hand blender
Heat again for another 35 minutes until brought to a simmer
Serve immediately, after cooling (5-10 minutes)

Additional Notes: if desired:
Add 1 cup of any (diced) 100% certified organic, farm raised, grass fed "baked" lemon-pepper and Greek seasoned meat

ALL NATURAL GRAINS SOUP

DAY 13
(ALL NATURAL GRAINS SOUP)

Typically makes 4-6 servings and lasts a few days, but utilize a "Small" Boiler Pot or "Small Sized Crock-Pot" (for best results) for smaller portions to watch your weight, prevent over-eating and watch your sodium (salt) intake.

Main Ingredients:
Into a Small Boiler Pot
Add 3-4 cups of whole wheat lentils, 1 cup of roasted pumpkin seeds, 1 cup of bulgur and 1 cup of whole wheat barley, 2 tablespoons of capers

Add 1 cup of diced onion, Add 1 cup of diced green bell pepper, Add 1 cup of diced red bell pepper, Add 1 cup of corn, Add 1 cup of diced parsley, Add 1 cup of diced roma tomatoes (both yellow and red), Add 1 cup of diced cilantro, Add a dash of salt, Add 1/2 teaspoon of ground red pepper, Add a dash of pepper, Add 1 diced garlic clove, Add 1/2 teaspoon of thyme, Add 2 teaspoons of certified 100% organic extra-virgin olive oil, Add 4-5 cups of (purified) water (regular cold tap water is fine as well), Bring to a boil

Cook for a few hours
Cook until thoroughly heated and boiled
Serve immediately, after cooling (5-10 minutes)

Additional Notes: if desired:
Add 1 cup of any (diced) 100% certified organic, farm raised, grass fed "baked" lemon-pepper and Greek seasoned meat

VEGETABLE GARDEN
CARROT STEW

DAY 14
(VEGETABLE GARDEN CARROT STEW)

Typically makes 4-6 servings and lasts a few days, but utilize a "Small" Boiler Pot or "Small Sized Crock-Pot" (for best results) for smaller portions to watch your weight, prevent over-eating and watch your sodium (salt) intake.

Main Ingredients:
Into a Small Boiler Pot
Add 4-6 cups of peeled and diced Certified 100% organic (home grown is best) carrots

Add 1 cup of diced onion, Add 1 cup of diced green bell pepper, Add 1 cup of diced red bell pepper, Add 1 cup of corn, Add 1 cup of diced parsley, Add 1 cup of diced roma tomatoes (both yellow and red), Add 1 cup of diced celery, Add a dash of salt, Add 1/2 teaspoon of ground red pepper, Add a dash of pepper, Add 1 diced garlic clove, Add 1/2 teaspoon of thyme, Add 2 teaspoons of certified 100% organic extra-virgin olive oil, Add 4-5 cups of (purified) water (regular cold tap water is fine as well), Bring to a boil

Cook for a few hours
Cook until thoroughly heated and boiled
Serve immediately, after cooling (5-10 minutes)
After cooling (20 minutes), puree the stew with a hand blender
Heat again for another 35 minutes until brought to a simmer
Serve immediately, after cooling (5-10 minutes)

Additional Notes: if desired:
Add 1 cup of any (diced) 100% certified organic, farm raised, grass fed "baked" lemon-pepper and Greek seasoned meat

BEATS & CELERY SOUP

ALL NATURAL SOUPS & STEWS

DAY 15
(BEATS & CELERY SOUP)

Typically makes 4-6 servings and lasts a few days, but utilize a "Small" Boiler Pot or "Small Sized Crock-Pot" (for best results) for smaller portions to watch your weight, prevent over-eating and watch your sodium (salt) intake.

Main Ingredients:
Into a Small Boiler Pot
Add 3-4 diced (into small squares) organic beats and 3-4 diced stalks of organic celery

Add 1 cup of diced onion, Add 1 cup of diced green bell pepper, Add 1 cup of diced red bell pepper, Add 1 cup of corn, Add 1 cup of diced parsley, Add 1 cup of diced roma tomatoes (both yellow and red), Add 1 cup of diced celery, Add a dash of salt, Add 1/2 teaspoon of ground red pepper, Add a dash of pepper, Add 1 diced garlic clove, Add 1/2 teaspoon of thyme, Add 2 teaspoons of certified 100% organic extra-virgin olive oil, Add 4-5 cups of (purified) water (regular cold tap water is fine as well), Bring to a boil

Cook for a few hours
Cook until thoroughly heated and boiled
Serve immediately, after cooling (5-10 minutes)

Additional Notes: **if desired:**
Add 1 cup of any (diced) 100% certified organic, farm raised, grass fed "baked" lemon-pepper and Greek seasoned meat

FENNEL & ARTICHOKE STEW

DAY 16
(FENNEL & ARTICHOKE STEW)

Typically makes 4-6 servings and lasts a few days, but utilize a "Small" Boiler Pot or "Small Sized Crock-Pot" (for best results) for smaller portions to watch your weight, prevent over-eating and watch your sodium (salt) intake.

Main Ingredients:
Into a Small Boiler Pot
Add 3-4 diced (into small squares) fennel bulbs, halved, cored and thinly sliced and 1-2 cups of artichoke hearts

Add 1 cup of diced onion, Add 1 cup of diced green bell pepper, Add 1 cup of diced red bell pepper, Add 1 cup of corn, Add 1 cup of diced parsley, Add 1 cup of diced roma tomatoes (both yellow and red), Add 1 cup of diced celery, Add a dash of salt, Add 1/2 teaspoon of ground red pepper, Add a dash of pepper, Add 1 diced garlic clove, Add 1/2 teaspoon of thyme, Add 2 teaspoons of certified 100% organic extra-virgin olive oil, Add 4-5 cups of (purified) water (regular cold tap water is fine as well), Bring to a boil

Cook for a few hours
Cook until thoroughly heated and boiled
Serve immediately, after cooling (5-10 minutes)
After cooling (20 minutes), puree the stew with a hand blender
Heat again for another 35 minutes until brought to a simmer
Serve immediately, after cooling (5-10 minutes)

Additional Notes: **if desired:**
Add 1 cup of any (diced) 100% certified organic, farm raised, grass fed "baked" lemon-pepper and Greek seasoned meat

SUN-DRIED TOMATO
& AVOCADO SOUP

DAY 17
(SUN-DRIED TOMATO & AVOCADO SOUP)

Typically makes 4-6 servings and lasts a few days, but utilize a "Small" Boiler Pot or "Small Sized Crock-Pot" (for best results) for smaller portions to watch your weight, prevent over-eating and watch your sodium (salt) intake.

Main Ingredients:
Into a Small Boiler Pot
Add 6-8 cups of sun-dried tomatoes and 2-3 finely diced avocados (add in towards the end)

Add 1 cup of diced onion, Add 1 cup of diced green bell pepper, Add 1 cup of diced red bell pepper, Add 1 cup of corn, Add 1 cup of diced parsley, Add 1 cup of diced roma tomatoes (both yellow and red), Add 1 cup of diced celery, Add a dash of salt, Add 1/2 teaspoon of ground red pepper, Add a dash of pepper, Add 1 diced garlic clove, Add 1/2 teaspoon of thyme, Add 2 teaspoons of certified 100% organic extra-virgin olive oil, Add 4-5 cups of (purified) water (regular cold tap water is fine as well), Bring to a boil

Cook for a few hours
Cook until thoroughly heated and boiled
Serve immediately, after cooling (5-10 minutes)

Additional Notes: if desired:
Add 1 cup of any (diced) 100% certified organic, farm raised, grass fed "baked" lemon-pepper and Greek seasoned meat

BARLEY, EGGPLANT
& CHICK PEA STEW

DAY 18
(BARLEY, EGGPLANT & CHICK PEA STEW)

Typically makes 4-6 servings and lasts a few days, but utilize a "Small" Boiler Pot or "Small Sized Crock-Pot" (for best results) for smaller portions to watch your weight, prevent over-eating and watch your sodium (salt) intake.

Main Ingredients:
Into a Small Boiler Pot
Add 3-4 cups of organic barley, 2-3 finely diced purple organic eggplants and 2-3 cups of chickpeas (drained)

Add 1 cup of diced onion, Add 1 cup of diced green bell pepper, Add 1 cup of diced red bell pepper, Add 1 cup of corn, Add 1 cup of diced parsley, Add 1 cup of diced roma tomatoes (both yellow and red), Add 1 cup of diced celery, Add a dash of salt, Add 1/2 teaspoon of ground red pepper, Add a dash of pepper, Add 1 diced garlic clove, Add 1/2 teaspoon of thyme, Add 2 teaspoons of certified 100% organic extra-virgin olive oil, Add 4-5 cups of (purified) water (regular cold tap water is fine as well), Bring to a boil

Cook for a few hours
Cook until thoroughly heated and boiled
Serve immediately, after cooling (5-10 minutes)
After cooling (20 minutes), puree the stew with a hand blender
Heat again for another 35 minutes until brought to a simmer
Serve immediately, after cooling (5-10 minutes)

Additional Notes: if desired:
Add 1 cup of any (diced) 100% certified organic, farm raised, grass fed "baked" lemon-pepper and Greek seasoned meat

ASPARAGUS SOUP

DAY 19
(ASPARAGUS SOUP)

Typically makes 4-6 servings and lasts a few days, but utilize a "Small" Boiler Pot or "Small Sized Crock-Pot" (for best results) for smaller portions to watch your weight, prevent over-eating and watch your sodium (salt) intake.

Main Ingredients:
Into a Small Boiler Pot
Add 3-4 cups diced asparagus stalks

Add 1 cup of diced onion, Add 1 cup of diced green bell pepper, Add 1 cup of diced red bell pepper, Add 1 cup of corn, Add 1 cup of diced parsley, Add 1 cup of diced roma tomatoes (both yellow and red), Add 1 cup of diced celery, Add a dash of salt, Add 1/2 teaspoon of ground red pepper, Add a dash of pepper, Add 1 diced garlic clove, Add 1/2 teaspoon of thyme, Add 2 teaspoons of certified 100% organic extra-virgin olive oil, Add 4-5 cups of (purified) water (regular cold tap water is fine as well), Bring to a boil

Cook for a few hours
Cook until thoroughly heated and boiled
Serve immediately, after cooling (5-10 minutes)

Additional Notes: if desired:
Add 1 cup of any (diced) 100% certified organic, farm raised, grass fed "baked" lemon-pepper and Greek seasoned meat

KALE & PINTO BEAN STEW

DAY 20
(KALE & PINTO BEAN STEW)

Typically makes 4-6 servings and lasts a few days, but utilize a "Small" Boiler Pot or "Small Sized Crock-Pot" (for best results) for smaller portions to watch your weight, prevent over-eating and watch your sodium (salt) intake.

Main Ingredients:
Into a Small Boiler Pot
Add 3-4 cups of chopped organic kale and 2-3 cans of organic pinto beans

Add 1 cup of diced onion, Add 1 cup of diced green bell pepper, Add 1 cup of diced red bell pepper, Add 1 cup of corn, Add 1 cup of diced parsley, Add 1 cup of diced roma tomatoes (both yellow and red), Add 1 cup of diced celery, Add a dash of salt, Add 1/2 teaspoon of ground red pepper, Add cumin, Add the juice of 1 lime, Add 1 diced garlic clove, Add 1/2 teaspoon of thyme, Add 2 teaspoons of certified 100% organic extra-virgin olive oil, Add 4-5 cups of (purified) water (regular cold tap water is fine as well), Bring to a boil

Cook for a few hours
Cook until thoroughly heated and boiled
Serve immediately, after cooling (5-10 minutes)
After cooling (20 minutes), puree the stew with a hand blender
Heat again for another 35 minutes until brought to a simmer
Serve immediately, after cooling (5-10 minutes)

Additional Notes: if desired:
Add 1 cup of any (diced) 100% certified organic, farm raised, grass fed "baked" lemon-pepper and Greek seasoned meat

WHITE BEAN
& ROSEMARY SOUP

DAY 21
(WHITE BEAN & ROSEMARY SOUP)

Typically makes 4-6 servings and lasts a few days, but utilize a "Small" Boiler Pot or "Small Sized Crock-Pot" (for best results) for smaller portions to watch your weight, prevent over-eating and watch your sodium (salt) intake.

Main Ingredients:
Into a Small Boiler Pot
Add 3-4 cans of organic white beans and 2-3 tablespoons of finely diced rosemary

Add 1 cup of diced onion, Add 1 cup of diced green bell pepper, Add 1 cup of diced red bell pepper, Add 1 cup of corn, Add 1 cup of diced parsley, Add 1 cup of diced roma tomatoes (both yellow and red), Add 1 cup of diced celery, Add a dash of salt, Add 1/2 teaspoon of ground red pepper, Add a dash of pepper, Add 1 diced garlic clove, Add 1/2 teaspoon of thyme, Add 2 teaspoons of certified 100% organic extra-virgin olive oil, Add 4-5 cups of (purified) water (regular cold tap water is fine as well), Bring to a boil

Cook for a few hours
Cook until thoroughly heated and boiled
Serve immediately, after cooling (5-10 minutes)

Additional Notes: if desired:
Add 1 cup of any (diced) 100% certified organic, farm raised, grass fed "baked" lemon-pepper and Greek seasoned meat

CONGRATULATIONS ON YOUR NEW YOU!

Feel free to continue to use these soup and stew ideas to reward yourself once a month, during holidays or even on company retreats and family vacations for staying fit and healthy, on a dime, without compromising your weight management and health goals with unhealthy snacks.

Keep up the great work by continuing
on with my two newest books, "The 21 Day Smoothie Fast"
and the "21 Day Salad Fast"

ALL NATURAL SOUPS & STEWS

INDEX OF RECIPES

www.ingramcontent.com/pod-product-compliance
Lightning Source LLC
Chambersburg PA
CBHW071841090426
42811CB00035B/2300/J